The pH Balance Cookbook: Re-balance Your Body, Prevent Sickness, and Feel Fantastic with These 25 Recipes

Disclaimer and Terms of Use: Effort has been made to ensure that the information in this book is accurate and complete, however, the author and the publisher do not warrant the accuracy of the information, text and graphics contained within the book due to the rapidly changing nature of science, research, known and unknown facts and Internet. The Author and the publisher do not hold any responsibility for errors, omissions or contrary interpretation of the subject matter herein. This book is presented solely for motivational and informational purposes only.

Table of Contents

Alkaline Smoothies

Green pH Smoothie

Ingredients:

- ¾ C coconut water
- ½ C raw creamed coconut
- 2 C spinach
- 1 avocado, pitted and peeled
- ½ chopped cucumber
- 2 tsp. lime zest
- 2 limes, halved and peeled
- 20 to 25 drops Stevia
- salt to taste
- 1 tsp. minced ginger
- 1 ½ C ice

Directions:

I. Throw everything into your Bullet or Vitamix and set on high for about a minute, until creamy
II. Serve in four 8 oz. glasses

Carrot Juice

Ingredients:
- 3 carrots, chopped
- 6 kale leaves, chopped
- 2 celery sticks, chopped
- ¼ lemon juice
- 1 tsp. habanero hot sauce

Directions:

Add everything into your juicer and blend until smooth

Healthy Smoothie

Ingredients:
- 1 avocado
- 4 C baby spinach
- 1 C water
- lemon juice
- 1 cucumber, chopped
- 3 stems parsley
- mint
- 1" ginger
- ¼ C ice
- 1 tsp. Udo's oil

Directions:

I. Add everything into your food processor and blend until smooth
II. Add ice or water to modify the consistency to your desire

Peachy pH Smoothie

Ingredients:
- 1 peach, pitted
- 1 banana, peeled
- ¼ C baby spinach
- 1 tsp. agave
- 1 C coconut water

Directions:

Add everything in your blender or food processor and blend until smooth

Pineapple pH Smoothie

Ingredients:
- 2 C fresh spinach
- 1 ½ C almond milk
- ½ C coconut water
- 3 C fresh pineapple
- 2 T coconut flakes

Directions:

I.   Blend everything together in a food processor or blender until smooth and creamy
II.   Add in ice and blend a little more
III. Blend

Kale and Banana

Ingredients:
- 2 bananas
- 2 T hemp seed
- 1 bag frozen blueberries
- 2 ½ C water
- 5 leaves kale, chopped

Directions:

I.   Add everything into a blender and blend on high speed
II.   You can add water as needed for consistency

Pear Salad Smoothie

Ingredients:
- 1 banana
- 2 ½ pears
- 2 T hemp seeds
- 1 bag frozen raspberries
- 2 ½ C water
- bunch arugula lettuce
- 1 T Stevia

Directions:

Add everything to your blender and blend until smooth

Apple Weeds Smoothie

Ingredients:
- 1 bunch dandelions
- 1 lemon, peeled
- 2 apples
- 1 banana
- 2 tsp. flaxseed

Directions:

Add everything to your blender and blend until smooth

Carrot Ginger

Ingredients:
- 1 bunch carrots
- 1 avocado
- 1/2 lemon
- 1/3" ginger
- 1/4 tsp. salt
- 1/4 tsp. cayenne pepper

Directions:

I.   Add everything to your juicer and enough water to cover the vegetables
II.   Blend until smooth

Favorite Fruit pH Smoothie

Ingredients:
- 1 bunch kale
- 1 apple, cored
- 1 avocado, peeled
- 1 to 2 drops Stevia

Directions:

I.   Throw everything into your blender or food processor and add enough water to cover the fruit

II.   Blend until smooth and serve immediately

Soups

Garden Vegetable Soup

Ingredients:
- 2 carrots
- 1 zucchini
- 1 rib celery
- 1 C broccoli
- 3 stalks asparagus
- 1 onion, chopped
- 1 qt. water
- 5 T vegetable broth
- 2 tsp. salt

Directions:

I.   Add water, onion and vegetable broth to a saucepan and bring to a boil
II.   Chop the rest of your vegetables in a food processor or blender so that they are chunked
III.   When you get the water to a boil, go ahead and turn the stove off and add everything into the hot water, let them set over the heat (with the burner turned OFF) until the vegetables are soft
IV.   Remove from the heat and pour everything into the blender and blend until thick and creamy

Pumpkin Tomato

Ingredients:
- 1 qt. water
- 1 pint fresh tomatoes, diced
- 1 sweet pumpkin
- 5 sweet onions, chopped
- 1 T EVOO
- 2 tsp. salt
- cayenne pepper to taste

Directions:

I. Sauté the onions in a large pot with oil
II. Cut the pumpkin in half and scoop the insides into a pot with the onions
III. Throw in the tomatoes and water and cook for about 20 to 25 minutes
IV. Pour your soup mixture into blender or food processor and blend
V. Once it reaches the texture you are looking for, pour into serving bowls

Avocado Tomato Broth

Ingredients:
- 2 avocados
- 1 tomato, halved
- 1 celery stick, chopped
- 1 small onion, chopped
- lemon juice, 1 lemon
- 1 C water

Directions:

I. Scoop out the innards of the avocados and make sure all of your vegetables are chopped
II. Add everything into your blender or a food processor and blend until smooth
III. Serve cool

pH Carrot Soup

Ingredients:

- 2 lbs. carrots
- 2 oz. millet
- 4 C vegetable broth
- 2 yellow onions
- 1 T EVOO
- ¼ tsp. salt
- ¼ tsp. cayenne pepper
- 1 bunch parsley
- 1 bunch chives

Directions:

I. Chop your vegetables and make sure they are ready for cooking
II. Heat oil in your saucepan and add the onions, stir fry for 2 to 3 minutes; once they are tender, add in the carrots and stir fry for about 10 more minutes
III. Add in the broth, cover; add salt and pepper next, cook for another 25 to 30 minutes; you want the carrots to be soft and tender and remove from heat
IV. Puree the blend with a hand mixer and season to taste
V. Garnish with chives and parsley

Coconut Soup

Ingredients:
- 1 lb. cauliflower
- 1 1/4 C coconut milk
- 1 C water
- 2 T lime juice
- 1/3 C EVOO
- 1/2 C coriander leaves, chopped
- 1/4 tsp. cayenne pepper
- 1/4 tsp. pepper
- 1/4 C coconut chips

Directions:

I. Steam the cauliflower and once steamed, add the cauliflower to the coconut milk and water

II. Blend the three in your food processor or blender and blend until smooth

III. Add in the remaining ingredients and blend for 60 seconds

IV. Pour into serving bowls and garnish with coconut and coriander to taste

Salads

Backyard Garden Salad

Ingredients:
- 1 head romaine
- 2 tomatoes, chopped
- 2 carrots, shredded
- 1 red pepper, diced
- 1 green pepper, diced
- 1 cucumber, diced
- 1 red onion, thin slices

Citrus Dressing

- 1/3 C lemon juice
- 3/4 olive oil
- 1 tsp. garlic
- 1/2 tsp. oregano
- 1/4 tsp. rosemary
- 1 tsp. basil
- 1/2 tsp. cumin
- 1 pinch salt
- 1 pinch cayenne pepper

Directions:

I.   For the dressing: Add everything into your blender and blend until emulsified
II.   For the Salad: Add all your vegetables into a large salad bowl and mix, toss with clean hands
III. Pour the dressing (above recipe) over the salad and season to taste with salt, pepper or seeds

Alkaline Salad on the Go

Ingredients:
- 2 ripe avocados
- 8 oz. carrots
- 8 oz. broccoli
- ½ C scallions
- 1 tsp. salt

Directions:

Dice all of your vegetables into a salad bowl, toss and season to taste with salt

Avocado Coleslaw

Ingredients:

- ½ C red cabbage
- 2 carrots, shredded
- 1 tomato, chopped
- 1 small red onion, sliced
- 3 T parsley, chopped
- 1 avocado, skinned
- 3 ½ T EVOO
- lemon juice from one lemon

Directions:

I.   First, you want to be sure that your cabbage and carrots are shredded, the tomato is chopped; add them to a bowl with the thinly sliced onion

II.   Blend your avocado, EVOO and lemon juice in a separate bowl and once it's all really well combined, just pour it over the salad

Chinese Cucumber Salad

Ingredients:

- 1 lb. cucumber
- 2 T minced garlic
- 3 T sesame oil
- salt and pepper to taste

Directions:

I.   Start with the oil in a bowl and shake a little salt and pepper into the bowl, stir with a wooden spoon

II.   Add the minced garlic to the bowl and combine

III.   Halve the cucumbers and then slice them thinly

IV.   Add the slices into the bowl and toss with the ingredients already in there

V.   Let sit in fridge for 10 to 15 minutes to chill before serving

Wild Avocado and Garlic Salad

Ingredients:
- 1 avocado
- 1 bunch garlic (wild)
- 3 tomatoes
- 1 red bell pepper
- 2 T EVOO
- salt to taste
- 1 tsp. cayenne pepper

Directions:

I.   Peel and slice your avocado
II.   Chop the bell pepper and tomatoes
III.   Add everything that is prepared in a bowl and add in chopped garlic, which needs to be in fine chopped pieces, almost like being minced
IV.   Toss everything in a bowl and drizzle with olive oil
V.   Season with salt and pepper

pH Dressing, and Dips

Any Salad Dressing

Ingredients:
- 1 T minced garlic
- 1/4 tsp. salt
- 1/2 C chopped parsley
- 1/3 C chopped mint
- 1 1/2 tsp. cracked black pepper
- 1 lemon juiced
- 1/3 C EOO

Directions:

I. Add everything together in your blender or food processor and pulse

II. You can add 1 T flaxseed if you like a thicker dressing

III. This is a great way to contribute to your pH diet plan or as a garnish to any salad

Spinach Dip

Ingredients:
- 1 bunch baby spinach
- 1 avocado
- 1 C parsley
- 1 C dill
- 1 T tahini
- 1 T minced garlic

Directions:

I.   Add everything into your blender and mix until creamy
II.   Pour into veggie dip serving tray
III.   Season with salt and cracked black pepper to taste
IV.   Chill for 30 minutes to an hour before serving with chilled vegetables or chips

Flower Pesto

Ingredients:

- 1 4 oz. bag sunflower seeds (shelled)
- 1 red pepper
- 1 tomato
- 1 T minced garlic
- EVOO
- ¼ tsp. salt
- ¼ tsp. pepper

Directions:

I.   Soak the sunflower seeds for about an hour (these are the ones NOT in the shells, these need to be the salted, ready-to-eat seeds)
II. Add everything into your blender and pulse until creamy
III. Season with salt and pepper or any herbs and seasonings you prefer
IV. Great for pasta or garlic bread

Caesar Dressing pH Style

Ingredients:
- 1/3 C EVOO
- 1/2 C water
- 1 T miso
- 1/2 lemon, juice
- 2 dates (soaked for 12 to 24 hours prior)
- 1 T minced garlic
- 1 tsp. cayenne
- 1 tsp. salt

Directions:

I. Add everything into your blender and pulse until everything is emulsified
II. Season to taste
III. Store any unused dressing in airtight container in refrigerator

Spicy pH Salsa

Ingredients:
- 3 big boy tomatoes
- 2 green chilies
- 2 onion sprigs, chopped
- 2 sweet onions
- 1 ½ T minced garlic
- ½ C cilantro, chopped
- 1 tsp. cayenne pepper
- lime juice

Directions:

I.   Wash and pat dry the tomatoes and chilies and chop into fine pieces
II. Slice the onions into rings
III. Toss everything together in a medium size bowl and dump into your blender or food processor long enough to pulse to desired salsa consistency; if you want CHUNKY salsa, chop and toss, do not blend
IV. Serve warm or chilled